Ahmed Harbaoui

Management of neck pain in military athletes

Ahmed Harbaoui

Management of neck pain in military athletes

ScienciaScripts

Imprint

Cover image: www.ingimage.com

This book is a translation from the original published under ISBN 978-620-6-72533-6.

Publisher:
Sciencia Scripts
is a trademark of
Dodo Books Indian Ocean Ltd. and OmniScriptum S.R.L publishing group

120 High Road, East Finchley, London, N2 9ED, United Kingdom
Str. Armeneasca 28/1, office 1, Chisinau MD-2012, Republic of Moldova, Europe
Printed at: see last page
ISBN: 978-620-8-29746-6

Table of contents

List of figures :

List of tables :

INTRODUCTION

Cervicalgia is a common musculoskeletal problem with a lifetime prevalence ranging from 14% to 70% in the general population [1].

According to the Global Burden of Disease report, neck pain accounts for the fourth highest number of years lived with disability [2], and its direct and indirect economic costs have encouraged researchers to study the prevalence and risk factors of neck pain in the general population.

Although the prevalence of neck pain in athletes can be considered similar to that of the general population, their sport-specific injuries may put them at higher risk of neck pain.

Athletes spend more time in sports activities and experience higher mechanical loads on their spines. These musculoskeletal stresses can accumulate over years of participation in professional sports, from adolescence to adulthood, depending on the type, intensity, frequency and duration of sporting activities [3].

Numerous studies have investigated the prevalence of low back pain in athletes [4].

Since similar studies of neck pain in athletes are rare, some studies have examined the prevalence of neck pain in athletic populations. However, these studies may have methodological limitations [5].

The etiology of neck pain is multifactorial. Factors such as the nature of the profession, ageing and lack of physical exercise are key factors in their genesis.

There are few studies of neck pain in the military environment, particularly in the case of sportsmen and women, who are subjected to numerous repetitive strain injuries.

Studies on this condition in the Tunisian army are still fragmentary and non-existent for military athletes.

The aim of this work was:

- To estimate the degree of sports and professional handicap caused by neck pain in the Tunisian military sports population.
- Implement primary and secondary prevention measures against this disease.

METHODS

I-POPULATION ANALYZED

Our cross-sectional descriptive study was carried out using a self-questionnaire intended for a population of 35 military athletes selected from the Bardo sports education barracks in Tunis.

I-I Inclusion criteria

We included in our study all high-level military athletes who had suffered at least one episode of cervicalgia or cervicobrachial neuralgia during their career, either acute (less than 3 months) or chronic (more than 3 months).

I- I Exclusion criteria

Athletes who developed neck pain or cervicobrachial neuralgia after definitive cessation of sporting competition were excluded from this study.

II- Methods

For all athletes, we collected epidemiological, clinical and radiographic data.

II-I Epidemiological data

We analyzed, for each subject, data relating to personal history, age, sex, rank and professional activity, nature and duration of sporting activity and anthropometric parameters.

II-2 Anthropometric data

For all military personnel, we considered height, weight and calculated Body Mass Index (BMI).

II-3 Clinical data

We carried out a physical examination with emphasis on osteoarticular examination for all subjects considered.

II- 4 Radiographic data

Standard X-rays of the cervical spine were analyzed for each athlete. CT or MRI data of the cervical spine were also studied for some of them.

III- Statistical data analysis

The data collected were processed using Excel 2007. Frequencies were calculated using the automatic filter available in this software. All statistical calculations were performed using SPSS software (P-value and analysis of variance). Qualitative parameters were compared using a chi-square test. P values below 0.01 and 0.05 were considered statistically significant. For numbers less than 5, we used the Fisher test as a corrective factor.

RESULTS

I-DESCRIPTIVE STUDY

I-1 Epidemiological data

I-1-1 Age

The average age of the subjects was 34.2±7.7 years, with extremes ranging from 17 to 58 years.

The age groups most frequently encountered were between 25 and 40 (42%) (Figure 1).

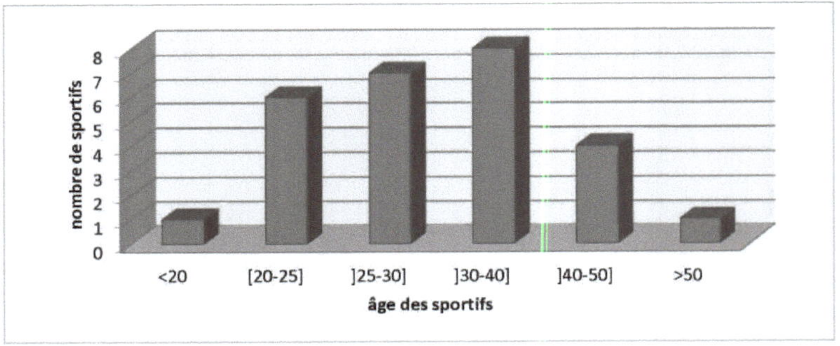

Figure 1: Distribution of athletes by age.

I-1-2 Gender

Males were predominant (88%). The sex ratio (M/F) was 5.7, with 29 men and 6 women (Figure 2).

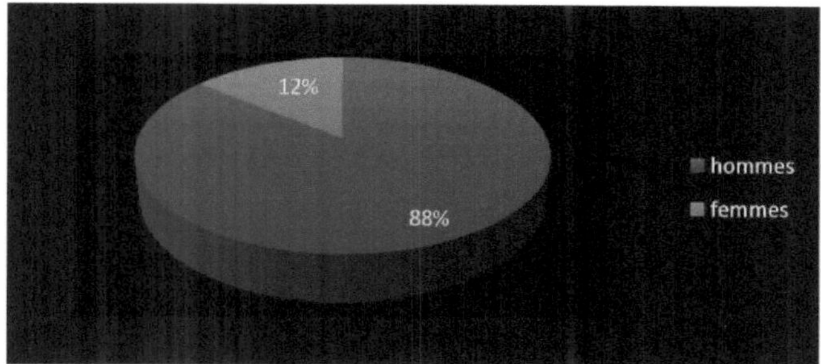

Figure 2: Distribution of athletes by gender.

I-1-3 Professional situation

The population comprised 3 officers (8%), 23 non-commissioned officers (66%) and 9 enlisted men (26%) (Figure 3).

Graduates held positions in administration (43%), sports coaching (39%) or sports (18%) (Figure 4).

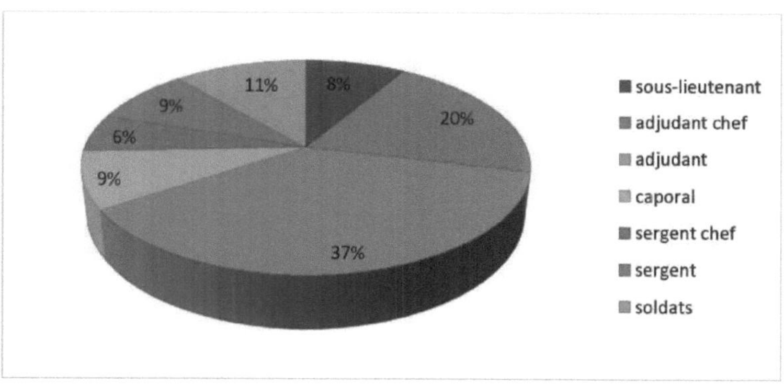

Figure 3: Breakdown of military sportsmen and women by rank.

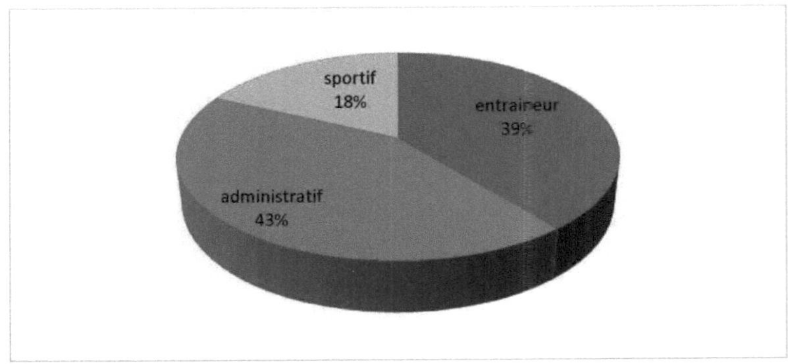

Figure 4: Distribution of military athletes by profession.

I-1-4 Duration of sports activities

The average age of military sportsmen and women in our population was 18.14±8.64 years. However, the majority (18 military athletes, or 54%) had been playing sports for less than 15 years (Figure 5).

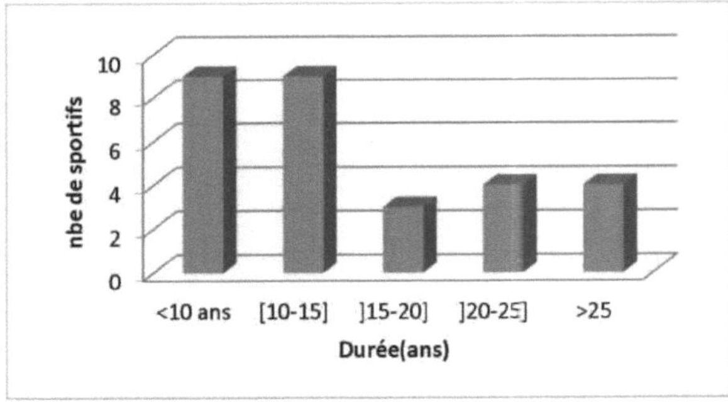

Figure 5: Distribution of military sportsmen and women by length of time spent in sport

I-1-5 Nature of sporting activity

In our study, 54% of the population took part in combat sports, boxing, judo and wrestling.

Ten (10) of the military athletes took part in athletics competitions.

In the female population, the 6 sportswomen each practiced different sports: athletics, judo, handball, shooting, swimming and wrestling (Figure 6).

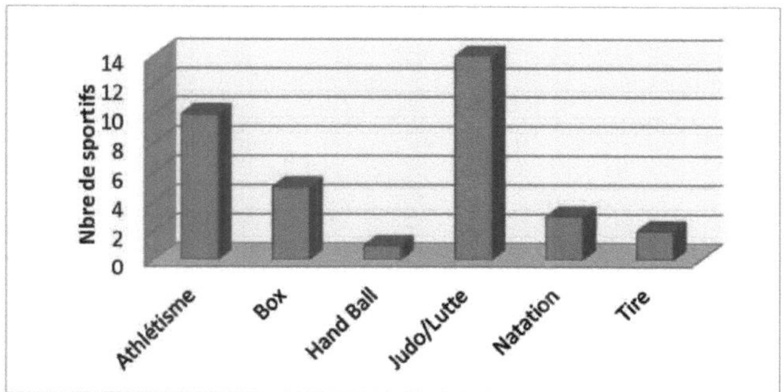

Figure 6: Distribution of athletes by type of sport.

I-1-6 Weekly and daily breakdowns of training sessions

The average number of training hours per week was 21±1.08 (Figure 7).

Training sessions were held every day of the week except Sunday.

The majority of our population, 24 athletes or 68%, had a daily training rhythm of 3 hours or less.

Two swimmers and a middle-distance runner trained 6 hours a day.

Four judokas did 4-hour sessions a day.

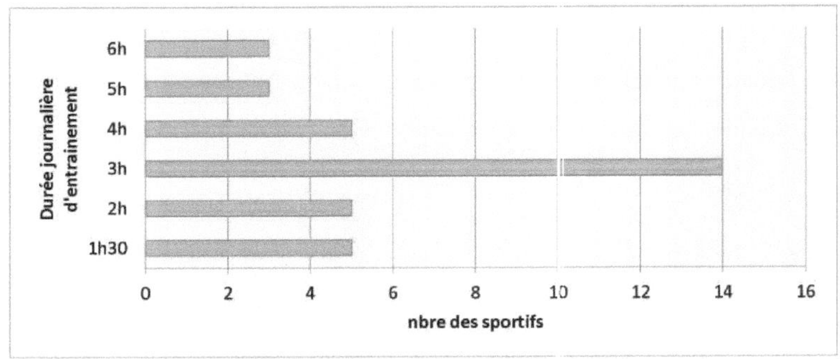

Figure 7: Variation in daily training time.

I-2 Clinical data

I-2-1 Body Mass Index (BMI)

Subjects' BMI ranged from 20 to 30, with a mean value of 24.64±4.43.

The majority of athletes (20 or 57.14%) had a BMI between 20 and 25 (Figure 8).

Seven (7) athletes (i.e. 20%), 3 judokas, 2 wrestlers and 2 athletes, were overweight (25≤BMI≤ 30).

Mean BMI was 24.64±4.43 with a range between 20 and 30.

57% of athletes had a BMI between 20 and 25.

Three judokas, two runners and two wrestlers were overweight.

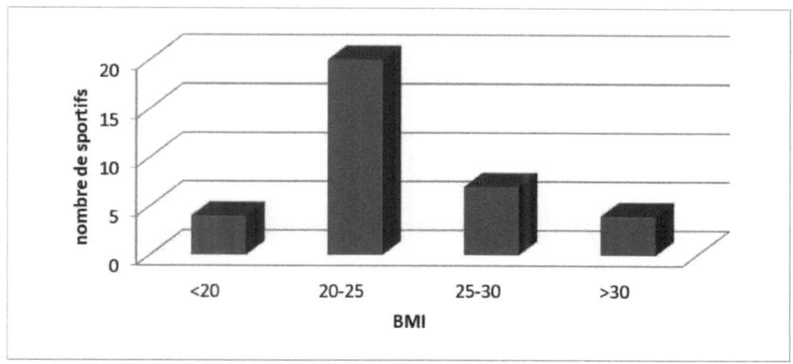

Figure 8: Distribution of athletes by BMI.

I-2-2 Characteristics and duration of symptoms

The duration of symptoms varied widely between the athletes in our study (from 1 to 96 months) (Figure 9).

The average duration was 40±30 months.

22.85% had symptoms that had been evolving for 4 years.

30 of the athletes had isolated mechanical neck pain.

5 of those questioned had associated cervicobrachial neuralgia

A post-traumatic context was found in 4 of our patients.

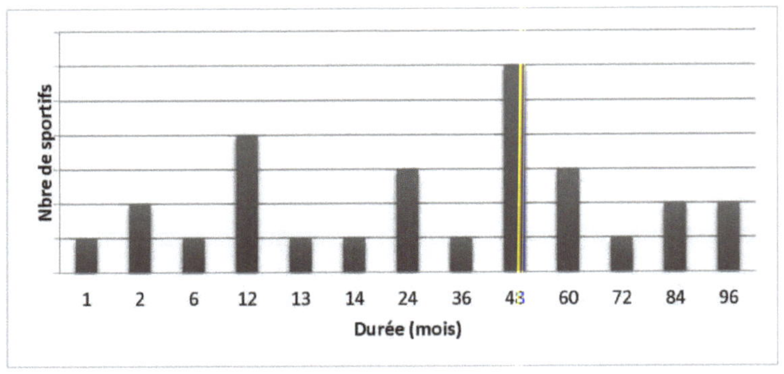

Figure 9: Distribution of athletes by duration of symptoms.

I-3 Pain assessment

26 of our patients presented with pain evolving in bursts, mainly during competitions.

5judokas, 2 athletes, 1 wrestler and 1 boxer, i.e. 9 athletes (25.71%) were suffering from pain at the time of the study.

I-4 Imaging data

Standard radiographs were taken in 20 patients: 12 had normal radiographs, 3 had straight cervical spine and 5 had osteoarthritis. (Figure 10).

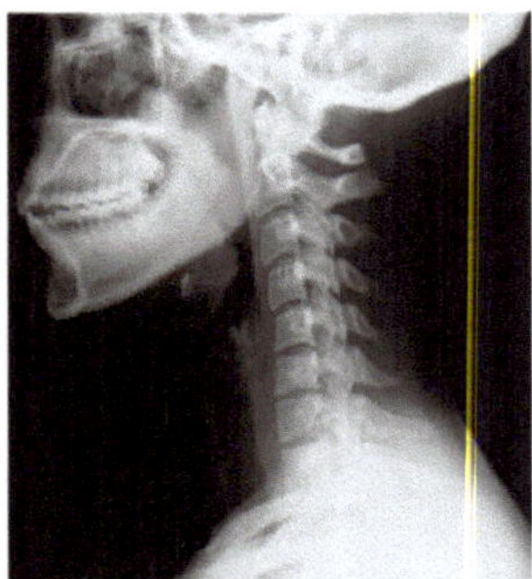

Figure 10: Standard X-ray of the cervical spine showing straightness.

A CT scan of the cervical spine was performed in the 4 patients with trauma and was unremarkable.

MRI of the cervical spine, performed in 6 patients, showed a herniated C4-C5 paramedian cervical disc in one patient, two patients had a herniated C5 C6 and one patient had a herniated C6 C7 (Figure 11).

MRI was normal in the other two patients.

Cervical disc herniation was observed in 1 wrestler, 3 judokas and one boxer.

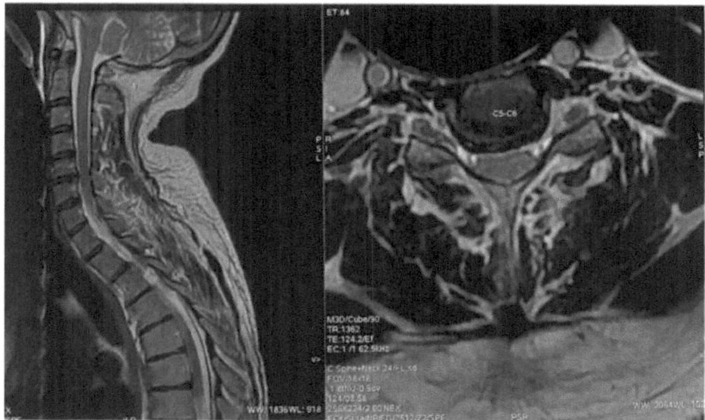

Figure 11: MRI of the cervical spine showing a C5 C6 hernia.

I-5 Therapeutic approach

Analgesic, anti-inflammatory and muscle relaxant treatment was administered to all patients in the series at the time of symptoms.

Treatment duration varied from 2 days to 1 month, depending on the severity of the attack.

Other therapeutic modalities have also been used:

- 16 patients (45.71%) underwent cervical rehabilitation
- 7 athletes (20%) wore a cervical collar
- 3 athletes (8.57%): 2 wrestlers and one boxer, were treated surgically with an anterior cervical approach and arthrodesis of the stage with the symptomatic herniated disc. All three patients had a favourable outcome, resuming sport after 6 months.

I-6 Impact of neck pain on work

16 patients (45.71%) were exempted from activities involving shaking, heavy lifting, prolonged standing or sitting for a total of 2 years. The other patients continued to exercise their professions normally.

I-7 Impact of neck pain on sporting activity

The impact of neck pain on sporting activities varied: 18 patients (51.42%) continued their sporting activities without any reduction in performance (Table 1). 5 runners, 3 boxers, 4 judokas, 2 wrestlers, 2 swimmers and 1 shooter had to stop practising their sport for a period ranging from one to six months.

The breakdown was as follows:

- 5 athletes (14.28%) had stopped physical activity for less than 10 days but had resumed the same level of activity.
- 4 athletes (11.42%) had to suspend competition for 1 month.
- 1 athlete (2.85%) stopped working for two months.
- 2 athletes (5.71%) suspended for 3 months.
- 1 athlete (2.85%) stopped working for 6 months.

- 4 athletes (11.42%): two judokas, one wrestler and one athlete stopped playing sport for good.

Table I: Impact of neck pain on sporting activity.

Downtime	Number of athletes
No stop	18
Less than 10 days	5
One month	4
Two months	1
Three months	2
Six months	1
Final stop	4

II-Correlations between the various neck pain parameters analyzed

The analysis of correlations between the duration of sporting activity and the various parameters did not take into account the type of activity, given the small number of cases for each discipline.

II-1 Duration of sporting activity and duration of symptoms

A statistically significant relationship was found between the duration of sporting activity and the duration of symptoms (P= 0.02) (Table 2).

II-2 Duration of sports activities and type of symptoms

There was no significant relationship between isolated neck pain and the presence of associated cervicobrachial neuralgia (P=0.67).

II-3 Duration of sports activities and duration of prescribed sick leave

There was no statistically significant correlation between these two elements (P=0.76) despite the wide variation in rest duration (1 to 6 months).

II-4 Duration of sports activities and duration of physiotherapy

The period of physiotherapy prescribed was not related to the overall duration of sporting activity (P=0.53).

Table II: Correlation between duration of sport and various neck pain parameters.

	X 2	P
Duration of symptoms	0,41	0,02
Type of symptoms	0,08	0,67
Duration of sick leave	0,06	0,76
Duration of physiotherapy	0,12	0,53

II-5 Correlations between weekly training duration and type and duration of symptoms

This analysis was based on the 35 individuals, without taking into account the type of activity, given the low numbers in each discipline.

There was no statistically significant relationship between training duration (in hours per week) and type (P=0.53) or duration of symptoms (P=0.30) (Table 3).

Table III: Correlation of weekly training duration with symptom type and duration.

	X 2	P
Type of symptoms	0,12	0,53
Duration of symptoms	-0,2	0,30

II-6 Correlations between type of sport and surgery

The three patients who underwent surgery practiced contact sports, boxing and wrestling.

II-7 Correlations between duration of neck pain and duration of occupational rest

This analysis, carried out on all athletes, showed a highly significant correlation between the duration of rest and the duration of neck pain ($p<0.001$), regardless of the type of sport practiced (Table 5).

Table IV: Correlation between duration of neck pain and duration of occupational rest.

	X2	P
Rest period	0,67	<0,001

DISCUSSION

Playing high-level sport (often at an early age and with intensive training) leads to numerous cervical injuries, particularly during hyperextension and rotation movements.

Leisure sport, on the other hand, seems to have a protective effect on the prevalence of this condition if it is not long and intensive and preceded by an appropriate warm-up [6].

In the military, the spine is subjected to numerous traumas and microtraumas during activities that often exceed their physical capacity (frequent carrying of heavy loads, driving off-road vehicles, parachute jumping, hand-to-hand combat), decompensating previously asymptomatic spinal statics anomalies.

What's more, the repercussions of this symptomatology within units are considerable in terms of downtime (sick leave in particular), operational inaptitude and healthcare costs.

In Tunisia, only one study [7] has looked at low back pain in the military, but no study has looked at neck pain.

No studies have been carried out on military personnel involved in high-level sports.

Our preliminary study is an essential step towards providing information on the extent of this condition in this population.

I-Evidence of neck pain

Most studies of neck pain in the military have been carried out in the USA and Europe.

These studies evaluated the incidence of neck pain in military aircraft pilots [8] and military personnel in administrative positions [9].

The average incidence of this condition in the general population was estimated at 15% in the USA and Canada [8]. Among military pilots, the incidence varied from 38% to 81%, depending on the study [8]. Among military personnel in administrative positions, the reported incidence of neck pain was e 65% [9].

In Tunisia, several epidemiological studies on neck pain have been carried out, mainly in hospitals, industry and schools. In the military, we are not aware of any study of this pathology.

In our study, which focused solely on a sample of military sportsmen with neck pain, this prevalence could not be accurately determined. The estimation of this parameter in our population can only be properly assessed by widening the sample and including non-symptomatic military sportsmen.

II-Risk factors for neck pain

Several risk factors for neck pain have been reported in both athletes and non-athletes. These include psychological factors such as stress and job dissatisfaction, but also insufficient or excessive physical exercise and poor posture [9].

Chronicity was more frequent in women. Social status, age and poor lifestyle also contributed to the onset of the condition.

In our study, we sought to correlate this condition with some of these factors.

II-1 Age of athletes

The population we studied was fairly young; the mean age of our patients was 34.2±7.7 years.

The most affected athletes were those aged between 30 and 40.

However, the correlation between this parameter and the occurrence of neck pain was not significant for the population we considered.

Young athletes are more prone to neck pain, due to repeated microtrauma to the growth plate of the vertebrae as a result of intensive training.

In a systematic review of the literature [5], analyzing the prevalence of neck pain in athletes, the average age was 29.

Elite athletes aged 18 to 27 were twice as likely to suffer from neck pain as controls [5].

The influence of age on neck pain may or may not be associated with the nature of the sport practised. Indeed, cross-sectional studies of adolescent athletes with an average age of 14 years found an association between the nature of the sport practised and the incidence of neck pain, which was 48.8% [10].

II-2 Influence of athletes' grade and functional position

Jobs involving the manual handling of heavy loads and those requiring prolonged postures or repeated flexion-extension movements with neck rotation are at high risk of neck pain [9].

The military profession, independently of sport, includes a combination of other specific risk factors, such as heavy lifting and carrying (75%), combat exercises (11%) and walking (10%), which trigger and aggravate neck pain

[8].

Physical and sporting activity, considered a protective factor against neck pain, may lose its effect during military service [5].

The chronicity of this condition can become a handicap to promotion to higher ranks. According to one study [11], 65% of servicemen suffering from neck pain were unable to reach the rank of officer or non-commissioned officer during their training.

In our study, warrant officers (37% of the population analyzed) were the most affected by neck pain, and most sportsmen and women (warrant officers or otherwise) held administrative positions (43%). Prolonged sitting and poor posture in these subjects would contribute to an increased risk of cervicalgia onset or aggravation.

However, according to our study, this association between grade-poste and neck pain was not significant, and the condition could have other origins.

II-3 Influence of Body Mass Index (BMI)

In both the general population and athletes, BMI is considered a determining factor in the occurrence of neck pain [12].

The mean BMI of our population was 24.64±4.43 indicating a slight tendency towards overweight.

This value was comparable to that reported in the series by Shariat et al [13], who found a significant association between BMI and the occurrence and intensity of neck pain.

Indeed, obese employees had a higher risk of developing symptoms, while being less likely to have these symptoms disappear than normal-weight employees. A large amount of adipose tissue around muscles and joints can restrict a person's movements, causing musculoskeletal tissue overload, which can lead to pain [14].

The effect of this factor on our population could therefore not be estimated, since the BMIs found did not differ significantly from the BMIs of non-athletes.

II-4 Influence of type of sport, weekly training and duration of sporting activity

The main risk factors for neck pain in athletes were often related to the age of onset of sporting activity, the age of the athlete and intensive practice of a single sport [5].

This risk increased in elite athletes [15]. Intensification of the training program was the most significant risk factor in the development of neck pain. Repetition of stereotyped movements and poorly adapted training also contributed to the onset of neck pain [6].

The longer the total period of sport practice, the greater the risk of intraspinal hernias and spondylolysis, which have been observed in subjects practising sport for more than four years [6].

In our study, the duration of sporting activity was 18.14±8.64 years, and training averaged 21±1.08 hours per week.

These two factors were not significantly related to the type of neck pain ($p=0.3$). Longer training time, at least in athletes, was a risk factor for neck pain [6].

Regarding the type of sport, the two most common types of neck pain reported in the literature were triathlon and cycling [6]. The level of pain reported by cyclists and triathletes was not similar, given that triathletes should theoretically have a more balanced load distribution between the three sports, and that the number of hours spent on the bike plays a major role in the symptoms of neck overuse injuries [6].

Driving, weightlifting, wrestling, running and ice hockey were also associated with neck pain [5].

In our work, we found that wrestlers - judoka (40%), athletes (28.57%) and boxers (14.28%) suffered the most neck pain.

However, the statistical correlation found in our work between neck pain and type of sport was not significant. Analysis of a larger sample of athletes in each sport category would enable us to clarify these results.

The occurrence of neck pain after cessation of sport must be taken into account in the protective or favourable role of sporting activity, although extra-sport activities take on greater importance here.

The prevalence of neck pain in former wrestlers was higher than in former weightlifters and an age-matched control group. Pain tolerance was better in athletes than in non-athletic controls [6].

III-Cervicalgia and anatomopathological lesions

The injury causing neck pain varies according to the age of the athlete and the type of sport practised.

The main mechanism of cervical injury is axial overload, i.e. a high compressive force applied to the top of the head [16].

The spectrum of cervical musculoskeletal injuries ranges from simple muscle or ligament sprains to bone and neurovascular injuries that can compromise central or peripheral nervous system function [16].

This mechanism is more dangerous when the neck is slightly flexed, as the spine moves out of its normal lordotic alignment, which doesn't allow the force to be distributed correctly over the thorax. Flexion places the cervical spine in a straight line, so the musculature cannot help absorb the force [16].

These lesions also differ according to the type of force and pre-existing degenerative lesions. Normal forces acting on a normal cervical spine can cause postural disorders, abnormal forces acting on a normal cervical spine and normal forces acting on a degenerative spine can cause sprains and ligament damage, while abnormal forces acting on a degenerative spine can cause more serious injuries [17].

Torg et al [18] reported that the cervical spine was injured when compressed between the body and the rapidly decelerating head. In the event of a fracture, if bone fragments or herniated disc material impinge on the spinal cord, neurological damage occurs. This mechanism was the main cause of cervical fractures, dislocations and quadriplegia.

A ligament sprain, one of the most common non-catastrophic injuries, may be associated with restricted spinal motion. A cervical sprain is produced by an overload of the muscle-tendon unit due to excessive forces exerted on the cervical spine [17].

Disc herniations are most often posterolateral, where the rate of curvature of the anulus is highest [17].

Excessive stress concentrations occur at these sites and can increase anular lesions, causing herniation of the nucleus pulposus, spurs of the anterior vertebral body, osteophytes of the posterior vertebral body and osteophytosis bars of the unco-vertebral joints with thickening of the yellow ligament and calcification of the posterior longitudinal ligament. All these degenerative changes can compromise normal function of the spine and bone [19].

MRI is useful for both early and late detection of disc degeneration [6]. In athletes, an association between the frequency and severity of neck pain (defined as cessation of sporting activity or training) and intraspinal herniations has been reported. However, a correlation between neck pain and signs of disc degeneration on MRI has not been observed [6].

In our study, 6 patients had herniated discs. Disc herniation was common in judokas (28.57%) and athletes (8.57%). The average age of these athletes was 34.2±7.7 years.

We were unable to identify a significant correlation between injury and the type of sport practised ($p=0.47$).

IV- Therapeutic management

In both military and civilian environments, neck pain often leads to over-medication and exaggeration of service-related causes [8,9]. Preventive measures combined with medical treatment can contribute to better disease management to meet professional and sporting imperatives.

V- Fighting neck pain

V-1 On a professional level

V-1-1 Professional selection

It enables us to select, at the time of recruitment, subjects likely to present a low probability of subsequent neck pain, with good musculature and the absence of spinal static disorders. However, a real difficulty in its application is linked to the high prevalence of neck pain at the age of enlistment, estimated in some studies at 50% at the age of 20.

V-1-2 Ergonomic measures

The ergonomic design of military vehicles and aircraft should minimize biomechanical constraints on personnel, in particular by reducing whole-body vibrations. Adapting workstations and work rhythms could also help.

Ergonomic studies specific to certain jobs assigned to athletes are essential.

Biomechanical and ergonomic studies were carried out to improve helmets, with the aim of modifying their center of gravity to improve load distribution and avoid axial overload and neck pain [8].

Foot orthoses, or "orthopedic inserts", have not been shown to be effective [8].

Finally, the effectiveness of technical lifting aids has never been demonstrated in controlled studies of good methodological quality [9].

V-1-3 Education and information

Information sessions in the workplace are available.

They should include anatomical explanations, learning how to handle loads, postures and strategies for adapting to neck pain.

The distribution of information booklets would be able to limit the frequency of recurrences and limit the transition to chronicity. The purpose of these booklets would be to provide reassuring information to patients, encourage them to maintain their professional and sporting activities, and avoid deconditioning during exercise.

V-2 Sports

Neck pain in top-level athletes is generally due to transient or long-lasting overload of the spine.

Treatment should be holistic: medical, sporting, psychological and environmental, not forgetting the prevention of recurrence.

V-2-1 Medical care

The medical treatment of neck pain in athletes does not differ from that of non-athletes. Medication is mainly used in the acute phase.

This is an essential element in avoiding the transition to chronicity.

Care must include :

- ✓ Effective symptomatic treatment is rapidly prescribed (analgesics, NSAIDs and relaxants).
- ✓ Bed rest should not be prescribed as a matter of course, but should only be authorized for short periods, and only in the event of very intense pain.

In our study, the overall duration of rest was not related (P=0.76) to the duration of sporting activity, but it was correlated with the duration of neck pain ($P<0.001$).

Our study should be extended by an annual analysis of these rest periods and the circumstances that led to their prescription.

V-2-2 Rehabilitation

Athletes suffering from neck pain may have deficits in mobility, muscle recruitment, endurance strength, postural stability, or oculomotor control [20].

The treatment of neck pain in athletes must take these deficits into account [21].

These deficits must be taken into account in the treatment of cervicalgia. The resulting exercise program must adequately prepare the athlete for the demands of his or her sport and a safe return to full participation [21].

1ère phase: crisis management

This phase is characterized by high pain intensity and irritability [21].

During this phase, the focus should be on slow, controlled and above all pain-free exercises designed to improve muscle coordination and proprioception [21].

2ème phase :

This phase is characterized by mild to moderate irritability, with a reduction in pain which is accentuated by exertion.

During this phase, muscular endurance should be improved through isometric exercises with low resistance. You should also continue to improve proprioception and postural stability exercises [21].

3ème phase: preventing recurrence

This phase is characterized by little or no irritability, with little or no neck pain on exertion.

During this phase, you need to strengthen your muscles with heavy loads and core muscles, not forgetting proprioception exercises [21].

Nelson et al [22] published a study in which they evaluated the outcome of aggressive, well-conducted rehabilitation for patients with neck pain for whom a surgical indication was given. They found that all patients improved after rehabilitation, and none required surgery.

V-2-3 Resuming training

It must be progressive, adapted to the athlete and the injury, with a thorough warm-up, without forgetting to correct the technopathy of the sport and to carry out a regular assessment of the athlete's physical condition.

V-3 Hygiene

Nutritional and water balance, weight and stress management, and personalized physical hygiene are all essential.

CONCLUSION

For many years now, neck pain has posed a considerable public health problem in terms of disability and time off work. The lifetime prevalence of this condition varies from 14% to 70% in the general population [1].

Few studies have been carried out on this condition in the military environment, and this is particularly true of military sportsmen and women, who are subjected to numerous cervical spine microtraumas in addition to their professional activities.

To our knowledge, there have been no studies of neck pain in Tunisian military sports.

In a population of 35 military sportsmen and women, we analyzed epidemiological data, types of neck pain symptoms and sporting activities (duration, nature, etc.).

The average age of our athletes was 34.2±7.7 years, with extremes ranging from 17 to 57 years. The age range between 30 and 40 was the most frequent. Males predominated. The sex ratio (M/F) was 5.66, with 29 men for 6 women. The subjects' BMI ranged from 20 to 30, with a mean value of 24.64±4.43. The majority of athletes (20 athletes or 57.14%) had a BMI between 20 and 25. 7 athletes (or 20%), 3 judokas, 2 wrestlers and 2 athletes, were overweight (25≤BMI≤ 30).

The ranks included 3 lieutenants, 7 chief warrant officers, 13 warrant officers, 3 corporals, 2 first sergeants, 3 sergeants and 4 privates. The ranks included administrative staff, sports coaches and athletes.

The average duration of sporting activity was 18.14±8.64 years. Over 50% of sportsmen and women had been practising for less than 20 years (25 sportsmen and women).

The sports practiced were diverse, including combat sports (wrestling, judo, boxing), athletics, swimming and shooting. Most athletes took part in combat sports (40%).

Our objective in this preliminary work was:

- Determine the degree of sporting and professional handicap caused by the condition.
- Implement primary and secondary prevention measures against neck pain.

Training was carried out on an almost daily basis (most of them resting on Sundays and Saturday afternoons). The average number of training hours was 21±1.08 per week, divided into 2 sessions of 3 hours per day on average.

5 athletes had developed cervicobrachial neuralgia, while the other 30 had cervicalgia only. Of the cervicalgias, 4 presented symptoms after cervical trauma.

The mean duration of neck pain was 40±30 months.

Standard radiography for 20 patients showed normal imaging in 12, straight cervical spine in 3 and osteoarthritis in 5.

MRI of the lumbar spine was performed in 6 patients, and showed cervical disc herniation in 4.

All patients received treatment with analgesics, NSAIDs or muscle relaxants at the onset of cervicalgia or cervicobrachial neuralgia. The treatment period varied from 2 days to 1 month, depending on the severity of the attack. Other prescribed treatments varied: 16 patients (45.71%) in all sports underwent rehabilitation for an average duration of 4.07±3.57 months; 7 athletes wore a cervical collar; 3 athletes, 2 wrestlers and one athlete, underwent surgery with a good post-operative outcome.

The impact of neck pain on sporting activities varied: 18 patients (51.42%) continued their sporting activities without any reduction in performance. The remaining 17 sportsmen and women, including 5 athletes, 3 boxers, 4 judokas, 2 wrestlers, 2 swimmers and 1 shooter, had to stop their sport either temporarily (1 to 6 months) or permanently.

The correlation between duration of sporting activity and duration of neck pain was significant at 5% (P= 0.02), indicating the presence of a positive correlation between these two parameters.

The duration of sporting activity was not significantly associated with the type of neck pain (P=0.67).

There was also no statistical correlation between the duration of sporting activity and the duration of prescribed rest (P=0.76), despite the wide variation in rest duration (1 to 6 months). However, the overall duration of rest was influenced by the duration of neck pain (P<0.001).

The prescribed rehabilitation period was not related to the overall duration of sporting activity (P=0.53). The duration of weekly training was not significantly correlated with the type of sport (P=0.53) or the duration of symptoms (P=0.30).

The type of sport practised was not correlated with the nature of the injury on imaging (standard X-ray, CT scan, MRI) (P=0.47), the duration of neck pain (P=0.87) and the duration of rest (P=0.51).

Analysis of all the correlations between the various parameters associated with neck pain (epidemiological, clinical, occupational, etc.) should be continued on a large sample of military sportsmen and women in order to recommend prevention and treatment of this condition.

It is necessary to include civilian athletes of the same level in the sample to be able to decompose the effects of occupation from those of sport.

Because of their role and duties, military athletes have certain characteristics that differ from those of civilian athletes. Their care, to improve their sporting skills and preserve their professional activities, should be more specific than that for civilian athletes.

REFERENCES

1. Hoy DG, Protani M, De R, Buchbinder R. The epidemiology of neck pain. Best Pract Res Clin Rheumatol. 2010 Dec;24(6):783-92.

2. Vos T, Flaxman AD, Naghavi M, Lozano R, Michaud C, Ezzati M, et al. Years lived with disability (YLDs) for 1160 sequelae of 289 diseases and injuries 1990-2010: a systematic analysis for the Global Burden of Disease Study 2010. Lancet Lond Engl. 2012 Dec 15;380(9859):2163-96.

3. Trompeter K, Fett D, Platen P. Prevalence of Back Pain in Sports: A Systematic Review of the Literature. Sports Med Auckl NZ. 2017 Jun;47(6):1183-207.

4. Schmidt CP, Zwingenberger S, Walther A, Reuter U, Kasten P, Seifert J, et al. Prevalence of low back pain in adolescent athletes - an epidemiological investigation. Int J Sports Med. 2014 Jul;35(8):684-9.

5. Noormohammadpour P, Farahbakhsh F, Farahbakhsh F, Rostami M, Kordi R. Prevalence of Neck Pain among Athletes: A Systematic Review. Asian Spine J. 2018 Dec;12(6):1146-53.

6. Villavicencio AT, Hernández TD, Burneikiene S, Thramann J. Neck pain in multisport athletes. J Neurosurg Spine. 2007 Oct 1;7(4):408-13.

7. Ksibi I, Kessomtini W, Maaoui R, Bejaoui A, Rahali Khachlouf H. Effect of a functional spine restoration program in chronic low back pain military personnel. J Réadapt Médicale Prat Form En Médecine Phys Réadapt. 2015 Jun 1;35(2):62-8.

8. Night Vision Goggle-Induced Neck Pain in Military Helicopter Airc...: Ingenta Connect [Internet]. [cited 2023 Sep 30]. Available from: https://www.ingentaconnect.com/content/asma/asem/2015/00000086/0000 0001/art00011

9. De Loose V, Burnotte F, Cagnie B, Stevens V, Van Tiggelen D. Prevalence and Risk Factors of Neck Pain in Military Office Workers.

Mil Med. 2008 May 1;173(5):474-9.

10. Legault ÉP, Descarreaux M, Cantin V. Musculoskeletal symptoms in an adolescent athlete population: a comparative study. BMC Musculoskelet Disord. 2015 Aug 20;16:210.

11. Cohen SP, Kapoor SG, Nguyen C, Anderson-Barnes VC, Brown C, Schiffer D, et al. Neck Pain During Combat Operations: An Epidemiological Study Analyzing Clinical and Prognostic Factors. Spine. 2010 Apr 1;35(7):758.

12. Nilsen TIL, Holtermann A, Mork PJ. Physical exercise, body mass index, and risk of chronic pain in the low back and neck/shoulders: longitudinal data from the Nord-Trondelag Health Study. Am J Epidemiol. 2011 Aug 1;174(3):267-73.

13. Shariat A, Cardoso JR, Cleland JA, Danaee M, Ansari NN, Kargarfard M, et al. Prevalence rate of neck, shoulder and lower back pain in association with age, body mass index and gender among Malaysian office workers. Work. 2018 Jan 1;60(2):191-9.

14. Berg T van den, Elders L, Zwart B de, Burdorf A. The effects of work- related and individual factors on the work ability index: A systematic review. Occup Environ Med [Internet]. 2008 Nov 18 [cited 2023 Sep 30]; Available from: https://oem.bmj.com/content/early/2008/11/18/oem.2008.039883

15. Joaquim AF, Hsu WK, Patel AA. Cervical spine surgery in professional athletes: a systematic review. Neurosurg Focus. 2016 Apr 1;40(4):E10.

16. Bailes JE, Petschauer M, Guskiewicz KM, Marano G. Management of Cervical Spine Injuries in Athletes. J Athl Train. 2007;42(1):126-34.

17. Cole AJ, Farrell JP, Stratton SA. Cervical Spine Athletic Injuries: A Pain in the Neck. Phys Med Rehabil Clin N Am. 1994 Feb 1;5(1):37-68.

18. Torg JS, Vegso JJ, O'Neill MJ, Sennett B. The epidemiologic,

pathologic, biomechanical, and cinematographic analysis of football-induced cervical spine trauma. Am J Sports Med. 1990;18(1):50 -7.

19. Franson RC, Saal JS, Saal JA. Human disc phospholipase A2 is inflammatory. Spine. 1992 Jun;17(6 Suppl):S129-132.

20. Childs JD, Cleland JA, Elliott JM, Teyhen DS, Wainner RS, Whitman JM, et al. Neck pain: Clinical practice guidelines linked to the International Classification of Functioning, Disability, and Health from the Orthopedic Section of the American Physical Therapy Association. J Orthop Sports Phys Ther. 2008 Sep;38(9):A1-34.

21. Durall CJ. Therapeutic Exercise for Athletes With Nonspecific Neck Pain: A Current Concepts Review. Sports Health. 2012 Jul 1;4(4):293-301.

22. Nelson BW, Carpenter DM, Dreisinger TE, Mitchell M, Kelly CE, Wegner JA. Can spinal surgery be prevented by aggressive strengthening exercises? A prospective study of cervical and lumbar patients. Arch Phys Med Rehabil. 1999 Jan;80(1):20-5.

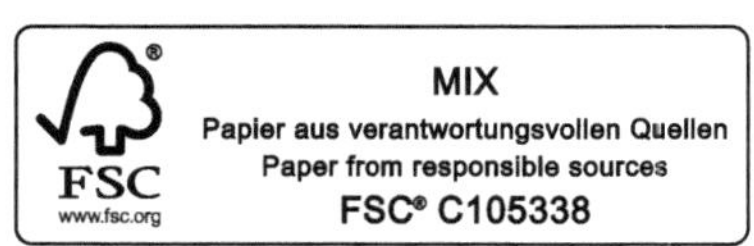

Printed by Books on Demand GmbH, Norderstedt / Germany